Air Fryer Toaster Oven Sweet Wonders

Tasty And Affordable Air Fryer Toaster Oven Recipes To Start Your Day with The Right Foot

AF256535

Cecil Braun

TABLE OF CONTENT

this book has been derived from various sources. Please consult a licensed professional before attempting any techniques outlined in this book.

By reading this document, the reader agrees that under no circumstances is the author responsible for any losses, direct or indirect, which are incurred as a result of the use of information contained within this document, including, but not limited to, — errors, omissions, or inaccuracies.

Mediterranean Egg Muffins with Ham

Preparation time: 15 minutes

Cooking time: 15 minutes

Servings: 6

INGREDIENTS:

- 9 Slices of thin cut deli ham
- 1/2 cup canned roasted red pepper, sliced + additional for garnish
- 1/3 cup fresh spinach, minced
- 1/4 cup feta cheese, crumbled
- 5 large eggs
- Pinch of salt
- Pinch of pepper
- 1 1/2 tbsp Pesto sauce
- Fresh basil for garnish

DIRECTIONS:

1. Preheat oven to 400 degrees F. Spray a muffin tin with cooking spray, generously.

Line each of the muffin tin with 1 ½ pieces of ham - making sure there aren't any holes for the egg mixture come out.

2. Place some of the roasted red pepper in the bottom of each muffin tin. Place 1 tbsp of minced spinach on top of each red pepper. Top the pepper and spinach off with a large 1/2 tbsp of crumbled feta cheese.

3. In a medium bowl, whisk together the eggs salt and pepper, divide the egg mixture evenly among the 6 muffin tins.

4. Bake for 15 to 17 minutes until the eggs are puffy and set. Remove each cup from the muffin tin. Allow to cool completely

5. Distribute the muffins among the containers, store in the fridge for 2 - 3days or in the freezer for 3 months.

NUTRITION: Calories: 109 Carbs: 2g Fat: 6g Protein: 9g

Quinoa Bake with Banana

Preparation time: 15 minutes

Cooking time: 1 hour & 10 minutes

Servings: 8

INGREDIENTS:

- 3 cups medium over-ripe Bananas, mashed
- 1/4 cup molasses
- 1/4 cup pure maple syrup
- 1 tbsp cinnamon
- 2 tsp raw vanilla extract
- 1 tsp ground ginger
- 1 tsp ground cloves
- 1/2 tsp ground allspice
- 1/2 tsp salt
- 1 cup quinoa, uncooked
- 2 1/2 cups unsweetened vanilla almond milk
- 1/4 cup slivered almonds

DIRECTIONS:

1. In the bottom of a 2 1/2-3-quart casserole dish, mix together the mashed banana, maple syrup, cinnamon, vanilla extract, ginger, cloves, allspice, molasses, and salt until well mixed.
2. Add in the quinoa, stir until the quinoa is evenly in the banana mixture. Whisk in the almond milk, mix until well combined, cover and refrigerate overnight or bake immediately.
3. Heat oven to 350 degrees F. Whisk the quinoa mixture making sure it doesn't settle to the bottom.
4. Cover the pan with tinfoil and bake until the liquid is absorbed, and the top of the quinoa is set, about 1 hour to 1 hour and 15 minutes.
5. Turn the oven to high broil, uncover the pan, sprinkle with sliced almonds, and lightly press them into the quinoa.
6. Broil until the almonds just turn golden brown, about 2-4 minutes, watching closely, as they burn quickly. Allow to cool

for 10 minutes then slice the quinoa bake

7. Distribute the quinoa bake among the containers, store in the fridge for 3-4 days.

NUTRITION: Calories: 213 Carbs: 41g Fat: 4g Protein: 5g

Italian Breakfast Sausage with Baby Potatoes and Vegetables

Preparation time: 15 minutes

Cooking time: 30 minutes

Servings: 4

INGREDIENTS:

- 1 lb. sweet Italian sausage links, sliced on the bias (diagonal)
- 2 cups baby potatoes, halved
- 2 cups broccoli florets
- 1 cup onions cut to 1-inch chunks
- 2 cups small mushrooms -half or quarter the large ones for uniform size
- 1 cup baby carrots
- 2 tbsp olive oil
- 1/2 tsp garlic powder
- 1/2 tsp Italian seasoning
- 1 tsp salt

- 1/2 tsp pepper

DIRECTIONS:

1. Preheat the oven to 400 degrees F. In a large bowl, add the baby potatoes, broccoli florets, onions, small mushrooms, and baby carrots.
2. Add in the olive oil, salt, pepper, garlic powder and Italian seasoning and toss to evenly coat. Spread the vegetables onto a sheet pan in one even layer.
3. Arrange the sausage slices on the pan over the vegetables. Bake for 30 minutes – make sure to sake halfway through to prevent sticking. Allow to cool.
4. Distribute the Italian sausages and vegetables among the containers and store in the fridge for 2-3 days

NUTRITION: Calories: 321 Fat: 16g Carbs: 23g Protein: 22g

Sun dried Tomatoes, Dill and Feta Omelet Casserole

Preparation time: 15 minutes

Cooking time: 40 minutes

Servings: 6

INGREDIENTS:

- 12 large eggs
- 2 cups whole milk
- 8 oz fresh spinach
- 2 cloves garlic, minced
- 12 oz artichoke salad with olives and peppers, drained and chopped
- 5 oz sun dried tomato feta cheese, crumbled
- 1 tbsp fresh chopped dill or 1 tsp dried dill
- 1 tsp dried oregano
- 1 tsp lemon pepper
- 1 tsp salt
- 4 tsp olive oil, divided

DIRECTIONS:

1. Preheat oven to 375 degrees F. Chop the fresh herbs and artichoke salad. In a skillet over medium heat, add 1 tbsp olive oil.
2. Sauté the spinach and garlic until wilted, about 3 minutes. Oil a 9x13 inch baking dish, layer the spinach and artichoke salad evenly in the dish
3. In a medium bowl, whisk together the eggs, milk, herbs, salt and lemon pepper. Pour the egg mixture over vegetables, sprinkle with feta cheese.
4. Bake in the center of the oven for 35-40 minutes until firm in the center. Allow to cool, slice a and distribute among the storage containers. Store for 2-3 days or freeze for 3 months

NUTRITION: Calories: 196 Carbohydrates: 5g Fat: 12g Protein: 10g

Mediterranean Breakfast Egg White Sandwich

Preparation time: 15 minutes

Cooking time: 30 minutes

Servings: 1

INGREDIENTS:

- 1 tsp vegan butter
- ¼ cup egg whites
- 1 tsp chopped fresh herbs such as parsley, basil, rosemary
- 1 whole grain seeded ciabatta roll
- 1 tbsp pesto
- 1-2 slices muenster cheese (or other cheese such as provolone, Monterey Jack, etc.)
- About ½ cup roasted tomatoes
- Salt, to taste
- Pepper, to taste
- Roasted Tomatoes:
- 10 oz grape tomatoes

- 1 tbsp extra virgin olive oil
- Kosher salt, to taste
- Coarse black pepper, to taste

DIRECTIONS:

1. In a small nonstick skillet over medium heat, melt the vegan butter. Pour in egg whites, season with salt and pepper, sprinkle with fresh herbs, cook for 3-4 minutes or until egg is done, flip once.
2. In the meantime, toast the ciabatta bread in toaster. Once done, spread both halves with pesto.
3. Place the egg on the bottom half of sandwich roll, folding if necessary, top with cheese, add the roasted tomatoes and top half of roll sandwich.
4. For the roasted tomatoes, preheat oven to 400 degrees F. Slice tomatoes in half lengthwise. Then place them onto a baking sheet and drizzle with the olive oil, toss to coat.
5. Season with salt and pepper and roast in oven for about 20 minutes, until the skin

appears wrinkled

NUTRITION: Calories: 458 Carbohydrates: 51g Fat: 0g Protein: 21g

Breakfast Taco Scramble

Preparation time: 15 minutes

Cooking time: 1 hour & 25 minutes

Servings: 4

INGREDIENTS:

- 8 large eggs, beaten
- 1/4 tsp seasoning salt
- 1 lb. 99% lean ground turkey
- 2 tbsp Greek seasoning
- 1/2 small onion, minced
- 2 tbsp bell pepper, minced
- 4 oz. can tomato sauce
- 1/4 cup water
- 1/4 cup chopped scallions or cilantro, for topping
- For the potatoes:
- 12 (1 lb.) baby gold or red potatoes, quartered
- 4 tsp olive oil
- 3/4 tsp salt
- 1/2 tsp garlic powder

- fresh black pepper, to taste

DIRECTIONS:

1. In a large bowl, beat the eggs, season with seasoning salt. Preheat the oven to 425 degrees F. Spray a 9x12 or large oval casserole dish with cooking oil.
2. Add the potatoes 1 tbsp oil, 3/4 teaspoon salt, garlic powder and black pepper and toss to coat. Bake for 45 minutes to 1 hour, tossing every 15 minutes.
3. In the meantime, brown the turkey in a large skillet over medium heat, breaking it up while it cooks. Once no longer pink, add in the Greek seasoning.
4. Add in the bell pepper, onion, tomato sauce and water, stir and cover, simmer on low for about 20 minutes. Spray a different skillet with nonstick spray over medium heat.
5. Once heated, add in the eggs seasoned with 1/4 tsp of salt and scramble for 2–3 minutes, or cook until it sets.

6. Distribute 3/4 cup turkey and 2/3 cup eggs and divide the potatoes in each storage container, store for 3-4 days.

NUTRITION: Calories: 450 Fat: 19g Carbs: 24.5g Protein: 46g

Blueberry Greek Yogurt Pancakes

Preparation time: 15 minutes

Cooking time: 15 minutes

Servings: 6

INGREDIENTS:

- 1 1/4 cup all-purpose flour
- 2 tsp baking powder
- 1 tsp baking soda
- 1/4 tsp salt
- 1/4 cup sugar
- 3 eggs
- 3 tbsp vegan butter unsalted, melted
- 1/2 cup milk
- 1 1/2 cups Greek yogurt plain, non-fat
- 1/2 cup blueberries optional
- Toppings:
- Greek yogurt
- Mixed berries – blueberries, raspberries and blackberries

DIRECTIONS:

1. In a large bowl, whisk together the flour, salt, baking powder and baking soda. In a separate bowl, whisk together butter, sugar, eggs, Greek yogurt, and milk until the mixture is smooth.

2. Then add in the Greek yogurt mixture from step to the dry mixture in step 1, mix to combine, allow the patter to sit for 20 minutes to get a smooth texture – if using blueberries fold them into the pancake batter.

3. Heat the pancake griddle, spray with non-stick butter spray or just brush with butter. Pour the batter, in 1/4 cupful's, onto the griddle.

4. Cook until the bubbles on top burst and create small holes, lift up the corners of the pancake to see if they're golden browned on the bottom

5. With a wide spatula, flip the pancake and cook on the other side until lightly browned. Serve.

NUTRITION: Calories: 258 Carbohydrates: 33g Fat: 8g Protein: 11

Cauliflower Fritters with Hummus

Preparation time: 15 minutes

Cooking time: 15 minutes

Servings: 4

INGREDIENTS:

- 2 (15 oz) cans chickpeas, divided
- 2 1/2 tbsp olive oil, divided, plus more for frying
- 1 cup onion, chopped, about 1/2 a small onion
- 2 tbsp garlic, minced
- 2 cups cauliflower, cut into small pieces, about 1/2 a large head
- 1/2 tsp salt
- black pepper
- Topping:
- Hummus, of choice
- Green onion, diced

DIRECTIONS:

1. Preheat oven to 400°F. Rinse and drain 1 can of the chickpeas, place them on a paper towel to dry off well.
2. Then place the chickpeas into a large bowl, removing the loose skins that come off, and toss with 1 tbsp of olive oil, spread the chickpeas onto a large pan and sprinkle with salt and pepper.
3. Bake for 20 minutes, then stir, and then bake an additional 5-10 minutes until very crispy.
4. Once the chickpeas are roasted, transfer them to a large food processor and process until broken down and crumble - Don't over process them and turn it into flour, as you need to have some texture. Place the mixture into a small bowl, set aside.
5. In a large pan over medium-high heat, add the remaining 1 1/2 tbsp of olive oil. Once heated, add in the onion and garlic, cook until lightly golden brown, about 2

minutes.

6. Then add in the chopped cauliflower, cook for an additional 2 minutes, until the cauliflower is golden.

7. Turn the heat down to low and cover the pan, cook until the cauliflower is fork tender and the onions are golden brown and caramelized, stirring often, about 3-5 minutes.

8. Transfer the cauliflower mixture to the food processor, drain and rinse the remaining can of chickpeas and add them into the food processor, along with the salt and a pinch of pepper.

9. Blend until smooth, and the mixture starts to ball, stop to scrape down the sides as needed

10. Transfer the cauliflower mixture into a large bowl and add in 1/2 cup of the roasted chickpea crumbs, stir until well combined.

11. In a large bowl over medium heat, add in enough oil to lightly cover the bottom of

a large pan. Working in batches, cook the patties until golden brown, about 2-3 minutes, flip and cook again. Serve.

NUTRITION: Calories: 333 Carbohydrates: 45g Fat: 13g Protein: 14g

Overnight Berry Chia Oats

Preparation time: 15 minutes

Cooking time: 5 minutes

Servings: 1

INGREDIENTS:

- 1/2 cup Quaker Oats rolled oats
- 1/4 cup chia seeds
- 1 cup milk or water
- pinch of salt and cinnamon
- maple syrup, or a different sweetener, to taste
- 1 cup frozen berries of choice or smoothie leftovers
- Toppings:
- Yogurt
- Berries

DIRECTIONS:

1. In a jar with a lid, add the oats, seeds, milk, salt, and cinnamon, refrigerate overnight. On serving day, puree the

berries in a blender.

2. Stir the oats, add in the berry puree and top with yogurt and more berries, nuts, honey, or garnish of your choice. Enjoy!

NUTRITION: Calories: 405 Carbs: 65g Fat: 11g Protein: 17g

Raspberry Vanilla Smoothie

Preparation Time: 5 minutes

Cooking Time: 5 minutes

Servings: 2 cups

INGREDIENTS:

- 1 cup frozen raspberries
- 6-ounce container of vanilla Greek yogurt
- ½ cup of unsweetened vanilla almond milk

DIRECTIONS:

1. Take all of your ingredients and place them in a blender. Process until smooth and liquified.

NUTRITION: Calories: 155 Protein: 7 g Fat: 2 g Carbohydrates: 30 g

Blueberry Banana Protein Smoothie

Preparation Time : 5 minutes

Cooking Time: 5 minutes

Servings: 1

INGREDIENTS:

- ½ cup frozen and unsweetened blueberries
- ½ banana slices up
- ¾ cup plain nonfat Greek yogurt
- ¾ cup unsweetened vanilla almond milk
- 2 cups of ice cubes

DIRECTIONS:

1. Add all of the ingredients into a blender. Blend until smooth.

NUTRITION: Calories: 230 Protein: 19.1 g Fat: 2.6 g Carbohydrates: 32.9 g

Chocolate Banana Smoothie

Preparation Time: 5 minutes

Cooking Time: 0 minutes

Servings : 2

INGREDIENTS:

- 2 bananas, peeled
- 1 cup unsweetened almond milk, or skim milk
- 1 cup crushed ice
- 3 tablespoons unsweetened cocoa powder
- 3 tablespoons honey

DIRECTIONS:

1. In a blender, combine the bananas, almond milk, ice, cocoa powder, and honey. Blend until smooth.

NUTRITION: Calories: 219 Protein: 2g
Carbohydrates: 57g Fat: 2g

Moroccan Avocado Smoothie

Preparation Time: 5 minutes

Cooking Time: 0 minutes

Servings: 4

INGREDIENTS:

- 1 ripe avocado, peeled and pitted
- 1 overripe banana
- 1 cup almond milk, unsweetened
- 1 cup of ice

DIRECTIONS:

1. Place the avocado, banana, milk, and ice into your blender. Blend until smooth with no pieces of avocado remaining.

NUTRITION: Calories: 100 Protein: 1 g Fat: 6 g Carbohydrates: 11 g

Mango Pear Smoothie

Preparation Time: 5 minutes

Cooking Time : 0 minute

Servings: 1

INGREDIENTS:

- 2 ice cubes
- ½ cup Greek yogurt, plain
- ½ mango, peeled, pitted & chopped
- 1 cup kale, chopped
- 1 pear, ripe, cored & chopped

DIRECTIONS:

1. Take all ingredients and place them in your blender. Blend together until thick and smooth. Serve.

NUTRITION: Calories 350 Protein 40g Fats 12g Carbohydrates: 11 g

Mediterranean Smoothie

Preparation Time: 5 minutes

Cooking Time: 5 minutes

Servings: 2

INGREDIENTS:

- 2 cups of baby spinach
- 1 teaspoon fresh ginger root
- 1 frozen banana, pre-sliced
- 1 small mango
- ½ cup beet juice
- ½ cup of skim milk
- 4-6 ice cubes

DIRECTIONS:

1. Take all ingredients and place them in your blender. Blend together until thick and smooth. Serve.

NUTRITION: Calories: 168 Protein: 4 g Fat: 1 g Carbohydrates: 39 g

Fruit Smoothie

Preparation Time: 5 minutes

Cooking Time: 0 minutes

Servings: 2

INGREDIENTS:

- 2 cups blueberries (or any fresh or frozen fruit, cut into pieces if the fruit is large)
- 2 cups unsweetened almond milk
- 1 cup crushed ice
- ½ teaspoon ground ginger (or other dried ground spice such as turmeric, cinnamon, or nutmeg)

DIRECTIONS:

1. In a blender, combine the blueberries, almond milk, ice, and ginger. Blend until smooth.

NUTRITION: Calories: 125 Protein: 2g
Carbohydrates: 23g Fat: 4g

Strawberry-Rhubarb Smoothie

Preparation Time : 5 minutes

Cooking Time: 3 minutes

Servings: 1

INGREDIENTS:

- 1 rhubarb stalk, chopped
- 1 cup sliced fresh strawberries
- ½ cup plain Greek yogurt
- 2 tablespoons honey
- Pinch ground cinnamon
- 3 ice cubes

DIRECTIONS:

1. Place a small saucepan filled with water over high heat and bring to a boil. Add the rhubarb and boil for 3 minutes. Drain and transfer the rhubarb to a blender.
2. Add the strawberries, yogurt, honey, and cinnamon and pulse the mixture until it is

smooth. Add the ice and blend until thick, with no ice lumps remaining. Pour the smoothie into a glass and enjoy cold.
NUTRITION: Calories: 295 Fat: 8g Carbohydrates: 56g Protein: 6g

Chia-Pomegranate Smoothie

Preparation Time: 5 minutes

Cooking Time : 0 minutes

Servings: 2

INGREDIENTS:

- 1 cup pure pomegranate juice (no sugar added)
- 1 cup frozen berries
- 1 cup coarsely chopped kale
- 2 tablespoons chia seeds
- 3 Medjool dates, pitted and coarsely chopped
- Pinch ground cinnamon

DIRECTIONS:

1. In a blender, combine the pomegranate juice, berries, kale, chia seeds, dates, and cinnamon and pulse until smooth. Pour into glasses and serve.

NUTRITION: Calories: 275 Fat: 5g Carbohydrates: 59g Protein: 5g

Egg White Scramble with Cherry Tomatoes & Spinach

Preparation Time: 5 minutes

Cooking Time: 8-10 minutes

Servings: 4

INGREDIENTS:

- 1 tbsp. Olive oil
- 1 whole Egg
- 10 Egg whites
- ¼ tsp. Black pepper
- ½ tsp. Salt
- 1 garlic clove, minced
- 2 cups cherry tomatoes, halved
- 2 cups packed fresh baby spinach
- ½ cup Light cream or Half & Half
- ¼ cup finely grated parmesan cheese

DIRECTIONS:

1. Whisk the eggs, pepper, salt, and milk. Prepare a skillet using the med-high temperature setting. Toss in the garlic

when the pan is hot to sauté for approximately 30 seconds.

2. Pour in the tomatoes and spinach and continue to sauté it for one additional minute. The tomatoes should be softened, and the spinach wilted.

3. Add the egg mixture into the pan using the medium heat setting. Fold the egg gently as it cooks for about two to three minutes. Remove from the burner, and sprinkle with a sprinkle of cheese.

NUTRITION: Calories 142 Protein: 15g Fat: 2g Carbs 4g

Blueberry, Hazelnut, and Lemon Breakfast Grain Salad

Preparation Time: 5 minutes

Cooking Time: 10 minutes

Servings: 8

INGREDIENTS:

- 1 cup steel-cut oats
- 1 cup dry golden quinoa
- ½ cup dry millet
- 3 tbsps. olive oil, divided
- ¾ tsp salt
- 1 x 1" piece fresh ginger, peeled and cut into coins
- 2 large lemons, zest and juice
- ½ cup maple syrup
- 1 cup Greek yogurt
- ¼ tsp nutmeg

- 2 cups hazelnuts, roughly chopped and toasted
- 2 cups blueberries or mixed berries
- 4 ½ cups water

DIRECTIONS:

1. Grab a mesh strainer and add the oats, quinoa, and millet. Wash well then pop to one side. Find a 3-quart saucepan, add a tbsp of the oil, and pop over medium heat.
2. Add the grains and cook for 2-3 minutes to toast. Pour in the water, salt, ginger coins, and lemon zest. Bring to the boil then cover and turn down the heat. Leave to simmer for 20 minutes.
3. Turn off the heat and leave to sit for five minutes. Fluff with a fork, remove the ginger then leave to cool for at least an hour. Grab a large bowl and add the grains.
4. Take a medium bowl and add the remaining olive oil, lemon juice, maple syrup, yogurt, and nutmeg. Whisk well to combine. Pour this over the grains and stir

well.

5. Add the hazelnuts and blueberries, stir again then pop into the fridge overnight. Serve and enjoy.

NUTRITION: Calories 363 Fat: 11g Carbs: 60g Protein: 7g

Feta & Quinoa Egg Muffins

Preparation Time: 20 minutes

Cooking Time: 45-50 minutes

Servings: 12

INGREDIENTS:

- 1 cup cooked quinoa
- 2 cups baby spinach, chopped
- ½ cup Kalamata olives
- 1 cup tomatoes
- ½ cup white onion
- 1 tbsp. fresh oregano
- ½ tsp. salt
- 2 tsp.+ more for coating pans olive oil
- 8 eggs
- 1 cup crumbled feta cheese
- Also Needed: 12-cup muffin tin

DIRECTIONS:

1. Heat the oven to reach 350° F. Lightly grease the muffin tray cups with a spritz of cooking oil.

2. Prepare a skillet using the medium temperature setting and add the oil. When it's hot, toss in the onions to sauté for two minutes.

3. Dump the tomatoes into the skillet and sauté for one minute. Fold in the spinach and continue cooking until the leaves have wilted (1 min.).

4. Transfer the pot to the countertop and add the oregano and olives. Set it aside.

5. Crack the eggs into a mixing bowl, using an immersion stick blender to mix them thoroughly. Add the cooked veggies in with the rest of the fixings.

6. Stir until it's combined and scoop the mixture into the greased muffin cups. Set the timer to bake the muffins for 30 minutes until browned, and the muffins are set. Cool for about ten minutes. Serve.

NUTRITION: Calories: 295 Carbs: 3g Fat: 23g Protein: 19g

5-Minute Heirloom Tomato & Cucumber Toast

Preparation Time: 10 minutes

Cooking Time : 6-10 minutes

Servings: 1

INGREDIENTS:

- 1 small Heirloom tomato
- 1 Persian cucumber
- 1 tsp. Olive oil
- 1 pinch Oregano
- Kosher salt and pepper as desired
- 2 tsp. Low-fat whipped cream cheese
- 2 pieces Trader Joe's Whole Grain Crispbread or your choice
- 1 tsp. Balsamic glaze

DIRECTIONS:

1. Dice the cucumber and tomato. Combine all the fixings except for the cream cheese. Smear the cheese on the bread and add the mixture. Top it off with the

balsamic glaze and serve.

NUTRITION: Calories: 239 Carbs: 32g Fat: 11g
Protein: 7g

Garbanzo Bean Salad

Preparation Time: 10 minutes

Cooking Time: 0 minutes

Servings: 4

INGREDIENTS:

- 1 ½ cups cucumber, cubed
- 15 oz. canned garbanzo beans, drained and rinsed
- 3 oz. black olives, pitted and sliced
- 1 tomato, chopped
- ¼ cup red onion, chopped
- 5 cups salad greens
- A pinch of salt and black pepper
- ½ cup feta cheese, crumbled
- 3 tbsps. olive oil
- 1 tbsp. lemon juice
- ¼ cup parsley, chopped

DIRECTIONS:

1. In a salad bowl, combine the garbanzo beans with the cucumber, tomato, and the

rest of the ingredients except the cheese
and toss.

2. Divide the mix into small bowls, sprinkle
    the cheese on top, and serve for
    breakfast.

NUTRITION: Calories 268 Fat: 16g Carbs: 24g
Protein: 9g

Brown Rice Salad

Preparation Time: 10 minutes

Cooking Time: 0 minutes

Servings: 4

INGREDIENTS:

- 9 oz. brown rice, cooked
- 7 cups baby arugula
- 15 oz. canned garbanzo beans, drained and rinsed
- 4 oz. feta cheese, crumbled
- ¾ cup basil, chopped
- A pinch of salt and black pepper
- 2 tbsps. lemon juice
- ¼ tsp lemon zest, grated
- ¼ cup olive oil

DIRECTIONS:

1. In a salad bowl, combine the brown rice with the arugula, the beans, and the rest of the ingredients, toss and serve cold for breakfast.

NUTRITION : Calories 473 Fat: 22g Carbs: 53g
Protein: 13g

Greek Yogurt with Walnuts and Honey

Preparation Time: 5 Minutes

Cooking Time : 0 minutes

Servings: 4

INGREDIENTS:

- 4 cups Greek yogurt, fat-free, plain or vanilla
- ½ cup California walnuts, toasted, chopped
- 3 tbsps. honey or agave nectar
- Fresh fruit, chopped or granola, low-fat (both optional)

DIRECTIONS:

1. Spoon yogurt into 4 individual cups. Sprinkle 2 tbsps. of walnuts over each and drizzle 2 tsps. of honey over each. Top with fruit or granola, whichever is

preferred.

NUTRITION: Calories 300 Fat: 10g Carbs: 25g Protein: 29g

27.   Tahini Pine Nuts Toast

Preparation Time: 5 minutes

Cooking Time : 0 minutes

Servings: 2

INGREDIENTS:

- 2 whole-wheat bread slices, toasted
- 1 tsp. water
- 1 tbsp. tahini paste
- 2 tsps. feta cheese, crumbled
- Juice of ½ lemon
- 2 tsps. pine nuts
- A pinch of black pepper

DIRECTIONS:

1. In a bowl, mix the tahini with the water and the lemon juice, whisk well, and spread over the toasted bread slices. Top each serving with the remaining ingredients and serve for breakfast.

NUTRITION: Calories 142 Fat: 7.6g Carbs: 13.7g
Protein: 5.8g

Crispy Pineapple Rings

Preparation Time: 5 minutes

Cooking Time: 7 minutes

Serving: 6

- 1 cup rice milk

- $\frac{2}{3}$ cup flour

- ½ cup water

- ¼ cup unsweetened flaked coconut

- 4 tablespoons sugar

- ½ teaspoon baking soda

- ½ teaspoon baking powder

- ½ teaspoon vanilla essence

- ½ teaspoon ground cinnamon

- ¼ teaspoon ground anise star

- Pinch of kosher salt

- 1 medium pineapple, peeled and sliced

Directions:

1. In a large bowl, stir together all the ingredients except the pineapple.

2. Dip each pineapple slice into the batter until evenly coated.

3. Arrange the pineapple slices in the air fryer basket.

4. Put the air fryer basket on the baking pan and slide into Rack Position 2, select Air Fry, set temperature to 380ºF (193ºC), and set time to 7 minutes.

5. When cooking is complete, the pineapple rings should be golden brown.

6. Remove from the oven to a plate and cool for 5 minutes before serving.

Coconut Pineapple Sticks

Preparation Time: 10 minutes

Cooking Time: 10minutes

Serving: 4

Ingredients:

- ½ fresh pineapple, cut into sticks
- ¼ cup desiccated coconut

Directions:

1. Place the desiccated coconut on a plate and roll the pineapple sticks in the coconut until well coated.
2. Lay the pineapple sticks in the air fryer basket.
3. Put the air fryer basket on the baking pan and slide into Rack Position 2, select Air Fry, set temperature to 400°F (205°C), and set time to 10 minutes.
4. When cooking is complete, the pineapple sticks should be crisp-tender.
5. Serve warm.

Chocolate Cheesecake

Preparation Time: 5 minutes

Cooking Time: 18 minutes

Serving: 6

Ingredients:

Crust:

- ½ cup butter, melted
- ½ cup coconut flour
- 2tablespoons stevia
- Cooking spray

Topping:

- 4ounces (113 g) unsweetened baker's chocolate
- 1cup mascarpone cheese, at room temperature
- 1teaspoon vanilla extract
- 2drops peppermint extract

Directions:

1. Lightly coat the baking pan with cooking spray.

2. In a mixing bowl, whisk together the butter, flour, and stevia until well combined. Transfer the mixture to the prepared baking pan.

3. Slide the baking pan into Rack Position 1, select Convection Bake, set temperature to 350ºF (180ºC), and set time to 18 minutes.

4. When done, a toothpick inserted in the center should come out clean.

5. Remove the crust from the oven to a wire rack to cool.

6. Once cooled completely, place it in the freezer for 20 minutes.

7. When ready, combine all the ingredients for the topping in a small bowl and stir to incorporate.

8. Spread this topping over the crust and let it sit for another 15 minutes in the freezer.

9. Serve chilled.

Peanut Butter-Chocolate Bread Pudding

Preparation Time: 10 minutes

Cooking Time: 10 minutes

Serving: 8

Ingredients:

- 1egg
- egg yolk
- ¾ cup chocolate milk
- 3tablespoons brown sugar
- 3tablespoons peanut butter
- 2tablespoons cocoa powder
- 1teaspoon vanilla
- 5slices firm white bread, cubed
- Nonstick cooking spray

Directions:

1. Spritz the baking pan with nonstick cooking spray.

2. Whisk together the egg, egg yolk, chocolate milk, brown sugar, peanut butter, cocoa powder, and vanilla until well combined.

3. Fold in the bread cubes and stir to mix well. Allow the bread soak for 10 minutes.

4. When ready, transfer the egg mixture to the prepared baking pan.

5. Slide the baking pan into Rack Position 1, select Convection Bake, set temperature to 330ºF (166ºC), and set time to 10 minutes.

6. When done, the pudding should be just firm to the touch.

7. Serve at room temperature.

Creamy Orange Cake

Preparation time: 10 minutes

Cooking time: 32 minutes

Servings: 12

Ingredients:

- 6eggs

  - 1orange, peeled and cut into quarters

  - 1teaspoon vanilla extract

  - 1teaspoon baking powder

  - 9ounces flour

  - 2ounces sugar+ 2 tablespoons

  - 2tablespoons orange zest

  - 4ounces cream cheese

  - 4ounces yogurt

Directions:

1. In your food processor, pulse orange very well.

2. Add flour, 2 tablespoons sugar, eggs, baking powder, vanilla extract and pulse well again.

3. Transfer this into 2 spring form pans, introduce each in your fryer and cook at 330 degrees F for 16 minutes.

4. Meanwhile, in a bowl, mix cream cheese with orange zest, yogurt and the rest of the sugar and stir well.

5. Place one cake layer on a plate, add half of the cream cheese mix, add the other cake layer and top with the rest of the cream cheese mix.

6. Spread it well, slice and serve.

Nutrition: calories 200, fat 13, fiber 2, carbs 9, protein 8

Coconut Macaroons

Preparation time: 10 minutes

Cooking time: 8 minutes

Servings: 20

Ingredients:

- 2tablespoons sugar
- 4egg whites
- 2cup coconut, shredded
- 1teaspoon vanilla extract

Directions:

1. In a bowl, mix egg whites with stevia and beat using your mixer.

2. Add coconut and vanilla extract, whisk again, shape small balls out of this mix, introduce them in your air fryer and cook at 340 degrees F for 8 minutes.

3. Serve macaroons cold.

Nutrition: calories 55, fat 6, fiber 1, carbs 2, protein 1

Lime Cheesecake

Preparation time: 4 hours and 10 minutes

Cooking time: 4 minutes

Servings: 10

Ingredients:

- 2 tablespoons butter, melted
- 2 teaspoons sugar
- 4 ounces flour
- ¼ cup coconut, shredded

For the filling:

- 1 pound cream cheese
- Zest from 1 lime, grated
- Juice form 1 lime
- 2 cups hot water
- 2 sachets lime jelly

Directions:

1. In a bowl, mix coconut with flour, butter and sugar, stir well and press this on the

bottom of a pan that fits your air fryer.

2. Meanwhile, put the hot water in a bowl, add jelly sachets and stir until it dissolves.

3. Put cream cheese in a bowl, add jelly, lime juice and zest and whisk really well.

4. Add this over the crust, spread, introduce in the air fryer and cook at 300 degrees F for 4 minutes.

5. Keep in the fridge for 4 hours before serving.

Nutrition: calories 260, fat 23, fiber 2, carbs 5, protein 7

Coconut Granola

Preparation time: 10 minutes

Cooking time: 35 minutes

Servings: 4

Ingredients:

- 1 cup coconut, shredded
- ½ cup almonds
- ½ cup pecans, chopped
- 2 tablespoons sugar
- ½ cup pumpkin seeds
- ½ cup sunflower seeds
- 2 tablespoons sunflower oil
- 1 teaspoon nutmeg, ground
- 1 teaspoon apple pie spice mix

Directions:

1. In a bowl, mix almonds and pecans with pumpkin seeds, sunflower seeds, coconut, nutmeg and apple pie spice mix and stir

well.

2. Heat up a pan with the oil over medium heat, add sugar and stir well.

3. Pour this over nuts and coconut mix and stir well.

4. Spread this on a lined baking sheet that fits your air fryer, introduce in your air fryer and cook at 300 degrees F and bake for 25 minutes.

5. Leave your granola to cool down, cut and serve.

Nutrition: calories 322, fat 7, fiber 8, carbs 12, protein 7

Fruity Cobbler

Preparation time: 10 minutes

Cooking time: 25 minutes

Servings: 6

Ingredients:

- ¾ cup sugar

- 6 cups strawberries, halved

- 1/8 teaspoon baking powder

- 1 tablespoon lemon juice

- ½ cup flour

- A pinch of baking soda

- ½ cup water

- 3 and ½ tablespoon olive oil

- Cooking spray

Directions:

1. In a bowl, mix strawberries with half of sugar, sprinkle some flour, add lemon juice, whisk and pour into the baking dish that fits your air fryer and greased with cooking spray

2. In another bowl, mix flour with the rest of the sugar, baking powder and soda and stir well.

3. Add the olive oil and mix until the whole thing with your hands.

4. Add ½ cup water and spread over strawberries.

5. Introduce in the fryer at 355 degrees F and bake for 25 minutes.

6. Leave cobbler aside to cool down, slice and serve.

Nutrition: calories 221, fat 3, fiber 3, carbs 6, protein 9

Milk Tea Cake

Preparation time: 10 minutes

Cooking time: 35 minutes

Servings: 12

Ingredients:

- 6 tablespoons black tea powder
- 2 cups milk
- ½ cup butter
- 2 cups sugar
- 4 eggs
- 2 teaspoons vanilla extract
- ½ cup olive oil
- 3 and ½ cups flour
- 1 teaspoon baking soda
- 3 teaspoons baking powder

For the cream:

- 6 tablespoons honey

- •	4 cups sugar

- •	1 cup butter, soft

Directions:

1. Put the milk in a pot, heat up over medium heat, add tea, stir well, and take off heat and leave aside to cool down.

2. In a bowl, mix ½ cup butter with 2 cups sugar, eggs, vegetable oil, vanilla extract, baking powder, baking soda and 3 and ½ cups flour and stir everything really well.

3. Pour this into 2 greased round pans, introduce each in the fryer at 330 degrees F and bake for 25 minutes.

4. In a bowl, mix 1 cup butter with honey and 4 cups sugar and stir really well.

5. Arrange one cake on a platter, spread the cream all over, top with the other cake and keep in the fridge until you serve it.

6. Enjoy!

Nutrition: calories 200, fat 4, fiber 4, carbs 6, protein 2

Lemony Plum Cake

Preparation time: 1 hour and 20 minutes

Cooking time: 36 minutes

Servings: 8

Ingredients:

- 7 ounces flour

- 1 package dried yeast

- 1 ounce butter, soft

- 1 egg, whisked

- 5 tablespoons sugar

- 3 ounces warm milk

- 1 and ¾ pounds plums, pitted and cut into quarters

- Zest from 1 lemon, grated

- 1 ounce almond flakes

Directions:

1. In a bowl, mix yeast with butter, flour and 3 tablespoons sugar and stir well.

2. Add milk and egg and whisk for 4 minutes until your obtain a dough.

3. Arrange the dough in a spring form pan that fits your air fryer and which you've greased with some butter, cover and leave aside for 1 hour.

4. Arrange plumps on top of the butter, sprinkle the rest of the sugar, introduce in your air fryer at 350 degrees F, bake for 36 minutes, cool down, sprinkle almond flakes and lemon zest on top, slice and serve.

Nutrition: calories 192, fat 4, fiber 2, carbs 6, protein 7

Raisin Cookies

Preparation time: 10 minutes

Cooking time: 25 minutes

Servings: 36

Ingredients:

- 1 cup water
- 1 cup canned lentils, drained and mashed
- 1 cup white flour
- 1 teaspoon cinnamon powder
- 1 cup whole wheat flour
- 1 teaspoon baking powder
- ½ teaspoon nutmeg, ground
- 1 cup butter, soft
- ½ cup brown sugar
- ½ cup white sugar
- 1 egg
- 2 teaspoons almond extract

- •   1 cup raisins

- •   1 cup rolled oats

- •   1 cup coconut, unsweetened and shredded

Directions:

1. In a bowl, mix white and whole wheat flour with salt, cinnamon, baking powder and nutmeg and stir.

2. In a bowl, mix butter with white and brown sugar and stir using your kitchen mixer for 2 minutes.

3. Add egg, almond extract, lentils mix, flour mix, oats, raisins and coconut and stir everything well.

4. Scoop tablespoons of dough on a lined baking sheet that fits your air fryer, introduce them in the fryer and cook at 350 degrees F for 15 minutes.

5. Arrange cookies on a serving platter and serve

6. Enjoy!

Nutrition: calories 154, fat 2, fiber 2, carbs 4, protein 7

Lentils And Dates Brownies

Preparation time: 10 minutes

Cooking time: 15 minutes

Servings: 8

Ingredients:

- 28 ounces canned lentils, rinsed and drained
- 12 dates
- 1 tablespoon honey
- 1 banana, peeled and chopped
- ½ teaspoon baking soda
- 4 tablespoons almond butter
- 2 tablespoons cocoa powder

Directions:

1. In your food processor, mix lentils with butter, banana, cocoa, baking soda and honey and blend really well.

2. Add dates, pulse a few more times, pour this into a greased pan that fits your air

fryer, spread evenly, introduce in the fryer at 360 degrees F and bake for 15 minutes.

3. Take brownies mix out of the oven, cut, arrange on a platter and serve.

4. Enjoy!

Nutrition: calories 162, fat 4, fiber 2, carbs 3, protein 4

Applesauce Cupcakes

Preparation time: 10 minutes

Cooking time: 20 minutes

Servings: 4

Ingredients:

- 4 tablespoons butter
- 4 eggs
- ½ cup pure applesauce
- 2 teaspoons cinnamon powder
- 1 teaspoon vanilla extract
- ½ apple, cored and chopped
- 4 teaspoons maple syrup
- ¾ cup white flour
- ½ teaspoon baking powder

Directions:

1. Heat up a pan with the butter over medium heat, add applesauce, vanilla, eggs and maple syrup, stir, and take off

heat and leave aside to cool down.

2. Add flour, cinnamon, baking powder and apples, whisk, pour in a cupcake pan, introduce in your air fryer at 350 degrees F and bake for 20 minutes.

3. Leave cupcakes them to cool down, transfer to a platter and serve them.

4. Enjoy!

Nutrition: calories 150, fat 3, fiber 1, carbs 5, protein 4

Sweet Rhubarb Pie

Preparation time: 30 minutes

Cooking time: 45 minutes

Servings: 6

Ingredients:

- 1 and ¼ cups almond flour
- 8 tablespoons butter
- 5 tablespoons cold water
- 1 teaspoon sugar

For the filling:

- 3 cups rhubarb, chopped
- 3 tablespoons flour
- 1 and ½ cups sugar
- 2 eggs
- ½ teaspoon nutmeg, ground
- 1 tablespoon butter
- 2 tablespoons low fat milk

Directions:

1. In a bowl, mix 1 and ¼ cups flour with 1 teaspoon sugar, 8 tablespoons butter and cold water, stir and knead until you obtain dough.

2. Transfer dough to a floured working surface, shape a disk, flatten, wrap in plastic, keep in the fridge for about 30 minutes, roll and press on the bottom of a pie pan that fits your air fryer.

3. In a bowl, mix rhubarb with 1 and ½ cups sugar, nutmeg, 3 tablespoons flour and whisk.

4. In another bowl, whisk eggs with milk, add to rhubarb mix, pour the whole mix into the pie crust, introduce in your air fryer and cook at 390 degrees F for 45 minutes.

5. Cut and serve it cold.

6. Enjoy!

Nutrition: calories 200, fat 2, fiber 1, carbs 6, protein 3

Crispy Lemon Tart

Preparation time: 1 hour

Cooking time: 35 minutes

Servings: 6

Ingredients:

For the crust:

- 2 tablespoons sugar
- 2 cups white flour
- A pinch of salt
- 3 tablespoons ice water
- 12 tablespoons cold butter

For the filling:

- 2 eggs, whisked
- 1 and ¼ cup sugar
- 10 tablespoons melted and chilled butter
- Juice from 2 lemons
- Zest from 2 lemons, grated

Directions:

1. In a bowl, mix 2 cups flour with a pinch of salt and 2 tablespoons sugar and whisk.

2. Add 12 tablespoons butter and the water, knead until you obtain dough, shape a ball, wrap in foil and keep in the fridge for 1 hour.

3. Transfer dough to a floured surface, flatten it, arrange on the bottom of a tart pan, prick with a fork, keep in the fridge for 20 minutes, introduce in your air fryer at 360 degrees F and bake for 15 minutes.

4. In a bowl, mix 1 and ¼ cup sugar with eggs, 10 tablespoons butter, lemon juice and lemon zest and whisk very well.

5. Pour this into pie crust, spread evenly, introduce in the fryer and cook at 360 degrees F for 20 minutes.

6. Cut and serve it.

7. Enjoy!

Nutrition: calories 182, fat 4, fiber 1, carbs 2, protein 3

Special Brownies

Preparation Time: 10 minutes

Cooking Time: 17 Minutes

Servings: 4

Ingredients

- 1 egg
- 1/3 cup cocoa powder
- 1/3 cup sugar
- 7 tbsp. butter
- ½ tbsp. vanilla extract
- ¼ cup white flour
- ¼ cup walnuts
- ½ tbsp. baking powder
- 1 tbsp. peanut butter

Directions:

1. Warm pan with 6 tablespoons butter and the sugar over medium heat, turn, cook for 5 minutes, move to a bowl, put salt, egg, cocoa powder, vanilla extract, walnuts, baking powder and flour, turn mix properly and into a pan.

2. Mix peanut butter with one tablespoon butter in a bowl, heat in microwave for some seconds, turn properly and sprinkle brownies blend over.

3. Put in air fryer and bake at 320° F and bake for 17 minutes.

4. Allow brownies to cool, cut.

5. Serve.

Nutrition:

Calories: 1350 kcal.

Protein: 22.38 g

Fat: 110.25 g

Carbohydrates: 85.49 g

Blueberry Scones

Preparation Time: 10 minutes

Cooking Time: 10 Minutes

Servings: 4

Ingredients

- 1 cup white flour
- 1 cup blueberries
- 2 eggs
- ½ cup heavy cream
- ½ cup butter
- 5 tbsp. sugar
- 2 tbsp. vanilla extract
- 2 tbsp. baking powder

Direction:

1. Mix in flour, baking powder, salt and blueberries in a bowl and turn.

2. Mix heavy cream with vanilla extract, sugar, butter and eggs and turn properly.

3. Blend the 2 mixtures, squeeze till dough is ready, obtain 10 triangles from mix, put on baking sheet into air fryer and cook them at 320°F for 10 minutes.

4. Serve cold.

Nutrition:

Calories: 2220 kcal

Protein: 34.75 g

Fat: 135.74 g

Carbohydrates: 212.9 g

Ricotta And Lemon Cake

Preparation Time: 15 minutes

Cooking Time: 1 hr. 10 Minutes

Servings: 4

Ingredients

- 8 eggs
- 3 lbs. ricotta cheese
- ½ lb. sugar
- Zest from 1 lemon
- Zest from 1 orange
- Butter for the pan

Directions:

1. Mix in eggs with lemon sugar, orange zest and cheese, then turn properly.

2. Smear pan with some batter, spray ricotta mix, get in the fryer at 39° F and roast for 30 minutes.

3. Lessen heat at 380°F and roast for 40 minutes still.

4. Remove from oven, allow to cool.

5. Serve.

Nutrition:

Calories: 4286 kcal

Protein: 224.96 g

Fat: 253.74 g

Carbohydrates: 275.77 g

Cheesy Brussels Spring

Preparation Time: 10 minutes

Cooking Time: 8 Minutes

Servings: 4

Ingredients

- 1 pound Brussels sprouts
- Juice of 1 lemon
- Salt and black pepper
- 2 tbsp. butter
- 3 tbsp. parmesan

Directions

1. Get Brussels sprouts into air fryer, cook them at 350° F for 8 minutes and move them to a bowl.

2. Melt the butter over heated pan on medium heat, put lemon juice, pepper and salt, blend properly and add to Brussels sprouts.

3. Put in parmesan, toss till it melts

4. Serve.

Nutrition:

Calories: 484 kcal

Protein: 22.41 g

Fat: 25.41 g

Carbohydrates: 54.39 g

Sweet Baby Carrots Dish

Preparation Time: 10 minutes

Cooking Time: 10 Minutes

Servings: 4

Ingredients

- 2 cups baby carrots
- A pinch of salt and black pepper
- 1 tbsp. brown sugar
- ½ tbsp. butter

Directions

1. Blend baby carrots with butter, pepper, salt and sugar in a bowl, toss, put into air fryer and cook at 350° F for 10 minutes.

2. Share in plates.

3. Serve.

Nutrition:

Calories: 76 kcal

Protein: 1.09 g

Fat: 5.87 g

Carbohydrates: 5.91 g

Collard Green Mix

Preparation Time: 10 minutes

Cooking Time: 10 Minutes

Servings: 4

Ingredients

- 1 bunch collard greens
- 2 tbsp. olive oil
- 2 tbsp. tomato puree
- 1 yellow onion
- 3 garlic cloves
- Salt and black pepper
- 1 tbsp. balsamic
- 1 tbsp. sugar

Directions

1. Blend oil, vinegar, garlic, tomato puree and onion in a bowl and beat.

2. Put in salt, pepper, collard greens and sugar. Toss, get it into air fryer. Cook at 320° F for 10 minutes.

3. Share collard greens blend on plates

4. Serve.

Nutrition:

Calories: 328 kcal

Protein: 1.84 g

Fat: 27.26 g

Carbohydrates: 20.95 g

Honey Duck Breasts

Preparation Time: 10 minutes

Cooking Time: 27 Minutes

Servings: 2

Ingredients

- 1smoked duck breast
- 1tbsp. honey
- 1tsp. tomato paste
- 1tbsp. mustard
- ½ tsp. apple vinegar

Direction

1. Mix tomato paste with honey, vinegar and mustard, whisk well. Add duck breast, toss it to coat move it to air fryer and cook at 370 ° F for 15 minutes.

2. Remove duck breast out from fryer. Add to honey mix, toss and loop back to air fryer then cook at 370°F for 6 minutes more.

3. Divide on plates then serve with side salad.

Nutrition:

Calories: 563 kcal

Protein: 59.68 g

Fat: 26.59 g

Carbohydrates: 19.28 g

Chinese Duck Legs

Preparation Time: 10 minutes

Cooking Time: 27 Minutes

Servings: 2

Ingredients

- 2 duck legs
- 2 dried chilies
- 1 tbsp. olive oil
- 2-star anise
- 1 bunch spring onions
- 4 ginger slices
- 1 tbsp. oyster sauce
- 1 tbsp. soy sauce
- 1 tsp. sesame oil
- 14 oz. water
- 1 tbsp. rice wine

Direction:

1. Heat pan with oil over medium high heat, add star anise, chili, rice wine, sesame oil, ginger, oyster sauce, water and soy sauce. Stir and cook for 6 minutes.

2. Put duck legs and spring onions, toss to coat. Transfer to pan and put in air fryer and cook at 370° F for 30 minutes.

3. Divide on plates then serve.

Nutrition:

Calories: 649 kcal

Protein: 52.02 g

Fat: 43.54 g

Carbohydrates: 12.27 g

Salmon And Chives Vinaigrette

Preparation Time: 10 minutes

Cooking Time: 15 Minutes

Servings: 4

Ingredients

- 2 tbsp. dill
- 4 salmon fillets
- 2 tbsp. chives
- 1/3 cup maple syrup
- 1 tbsp. olive oil
- 3 tbsp. balsamic vinegar
- Salt and black pepper

Directions

1. Season salmon with pepper and salt, rub with oil, put in air fryer. Cook at 350°F for 8 minutes.

2. Heat small pot with vinegar over medium heat. Add maple syrup, dill and chives, stir then cook for 3 minutes.

3. Divide fish on plates with chives vinaigrette on top and serve.

Nutrition:

Calories: 493 kcal

Protein: 3.25 g

Fat: 15.67 g

Carbohydrates: 89.9 g

Roasted Cod And Prosciutto

Preparation Time: 10 minutes

Cooking Time: 10 Minutes

Servings: 4

Ingredients

- 1 tbsp. parsley
- 4 medium cod filets
- ¼ cup butter
- 2 garlic cloves
- 2 tbsp. lemon juice
- 3 tbsp. prosciutto
- 1 tsp. Dijon mustard
- 1 shallot
- Salt and black pepper

Directions

1. Mix mustard with garlic, butter, shallot, parsley, lemon juice, pepper and salt, prosciutto and whisk well.

2. Season salmon with pepper and salt. Spread prosciutto mix over, put in air fryer and cook at 390°F for 10 minutes.

3. Divide on plates then serve.

Nutrition:

Calories: 446 kcal

Protein: 1.94 g

Fat: 46.52 g

Carbohydrates: 9.11 g

Greek Yogurt with Fresh Berries, Honey and Nuts

Preparation time: 5 minutes

Cooking time: 0 minutes

Servings: 1

INGREDIENTS:

> 6 oz. nonfat plain Greek yogurt
> 1/2 cup fresh berries of your choice
> 1 tbsp .25 oz crushed walnuts
> 1 tbsp honey

DIRECTIONS:

1. In a jar with a lid, add the yogurt. Top with berries and a drizzle of honey. Top with the lid and store in the fridge for 2-3 days.

NUTRITION: Calories: 250 Carbs: 35 Fat: 4g
Protein: 19g

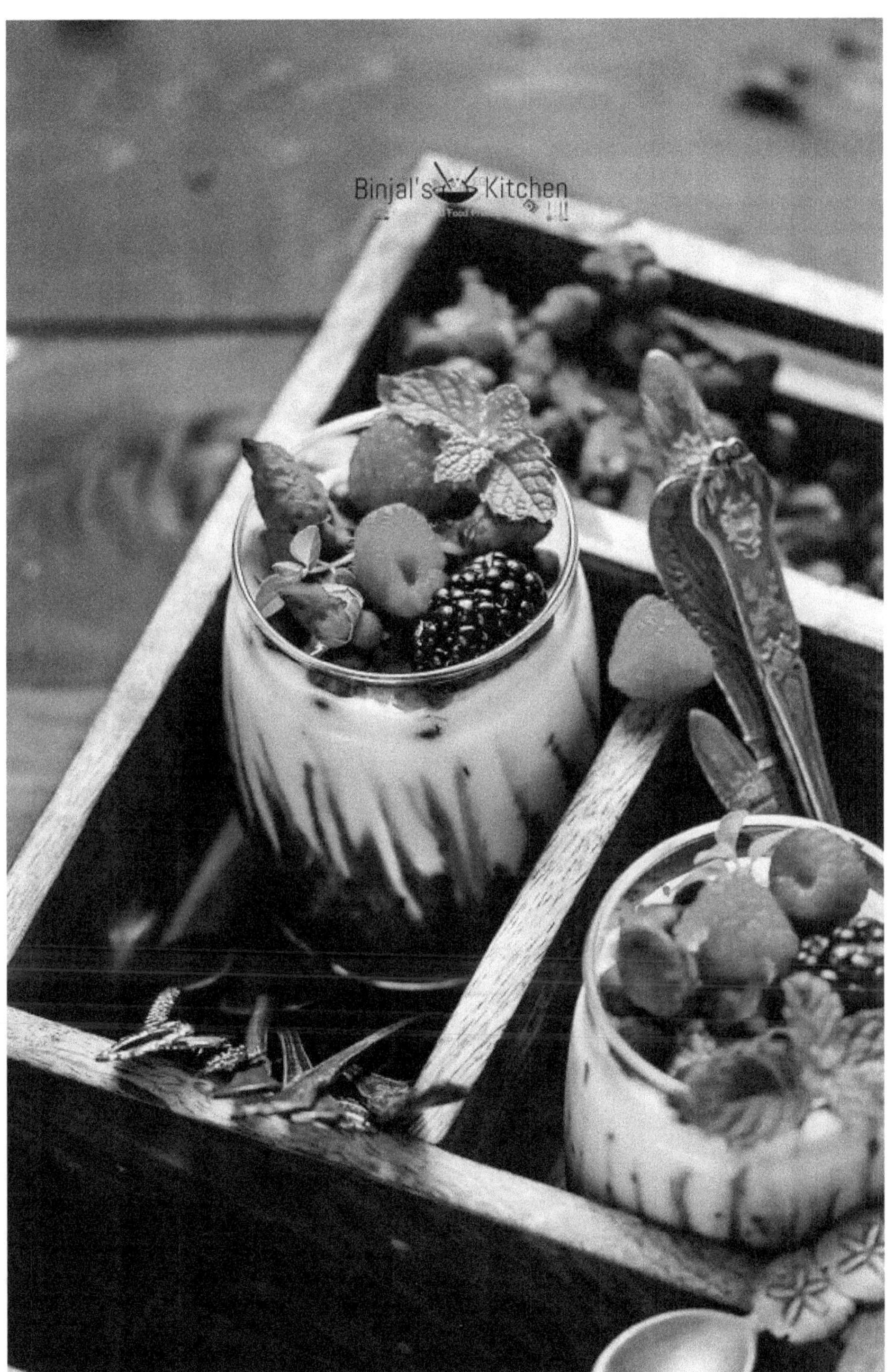